DAILY FOOD JOURNAL

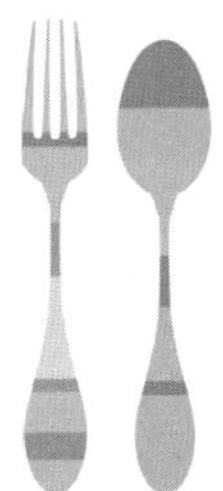

PETER PAUPER PRESS, INC.
WHITE PLAINS, NEW YORK

PETER PAUPER PRESS

Fine Books and Gifts Since 1928

Our Company

In 1928, at the age of twenty-two, Peter Beilenson began printing books on a small press in the basement of his parents' home in Larchmont, New York. Peter—and later, his wife, Edna—sought to create fine books that sold at "prices even a pauper could afford."

Today, still family owned and operated, Peter Pauper Press continues to honor our founders' legacy—and our customers' expectations—of beauty, quality, and value.

Designed by Heather Zschock

202 Mamaroneck Avenue
White Plains, NY 10601

ISBN 978-1-4413-1969-2
Printed in China

7

Visit us at www.peterpauper.com

You have a valuable tool in your hands that will help you achieve and maintain your optimal weight. Studies show that recording what we eat and how we exercise helps us lose up to 50 percent more weight. Writing down what we eat keeps us honest about our actual consumption, which helps us stay on track to attain our ideal weight goal. This guided notebook will help you track your caloric intake and expenditure by providing a place to record your daily foods and exercise.

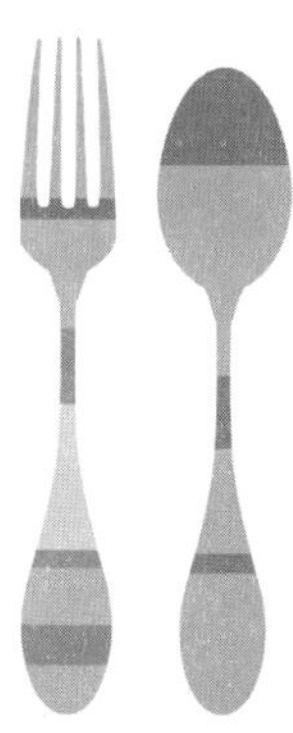

Here are a few tips to get you started:

- You cannot eat too many vegetables. Load up on the green, leafy kind and the orange and red ones. Let veggies fill you up with nutrients and fiber.
- Enjoy some fruit every day, too.
- Switch from highly processed, quickly digested carbs to complex carbs in whole grains.
- Go for lean proteins in grains, fish, fat-free dairy, eggs, poultry, and lean meat.
- Drink enough water to keep you hydrated.
- MOVE! Then move some more.
- Chew your food at least 20 to 30 times before you swallow.
- Think about what you're putting into your body before you eat.

Record notes about your personal progress on the last page.

DATE: Su Mo Tu We Th Fr Sa

Breakfast:	Amount	Calories (kcal)
	Total:	

Snack:	Amount	Calories (kcal)
	Total:	

Lunch:	Amount	Calories (kcal)
	Total:	

Snack:	Amount	Calories (kcal)
	Total:	
Dinner:	Amount	Calories (kcal)
	Total:	
Snack:	Amount	Calories (kcal)
	Total:	

Cups of Water: □□□□□□□□ **Servings of Fruits/Veggies:** □□□□□□□□

Exercise:	Duration	Calories (kcal) burned

DATE: Su Mo Tu We Th Fr Sa

Breakfast:	Amount	Calories (kcal)
	Total:	

Snack:	Amount	Calories (kcal)
	Total:	

Lunch:	Amount	Calories (kcal)
	Total:	

Snack:	Amount	Calories (kcal)
	Total:	
Dinner:	Amount	Calories (kcal)
	Total:	
Snack:	Amount	Calories (kcal)
	Total:	

Cups of Water: □□□□□□□□ **Servings of Fruits/Veggies:** □□□□□□□□

Exercise:	Duration	Calories (kcal) burned

DATE: Su Mo Tu We Th Fr Sa

Breakfast:	Amount	Calories (kcal)
	Total:	
Snack:	Amount	Calories (kcal)
	Total:	
Lunch:	Amount	Calories (kcal)
	Total:	

Snack:	Amount	Calories (kcal)
	Total:	

Dinner:	Amount	Calories (kcal)
	Total:	

Snack:	Amount	Calories (kcal)
	Total:	

Cups of Water: ☐☐☐☐☐☐☐☐ **Servings of Fruits/Veggies:** ☐☐☐☐☐☐☐☐

Exercise:	Duration	Calories (kcal) burned

DATE: Su Mo Tu We Th Fr Sa

Breakfast:	Amount	Calories (kcal)
	Total:	
Snack:	Amount	Calories (kcal)
	Total:	
Lunch:	Amount	Calories (kcal)
	Total:	

Snack:	Amount	Calories (kcal)
	Total:	

Dinner:	Amount	Calories (kcal)
	Total:	

Snack:	Amount	Calories (kcal)
	Total:	

Cups of Water: □□□□□□□□ **Servings of Fruits/Veggies:** □□□□□□□□

Exercise:	Duration	Calories (kcal) burned

DATE: Su Mo Tu We Th Fr Sa

Breakfast:	Amount	Calories (kcal)
	Total:	

Snack:	Amount	Calories (kcal)
	Total:	

Lunch:	Amount	Calories (kcal)
	Total:	

Snack:	Amount	Calories (kcal)
	Total:	

Dinner:	Amount	Calories (kcal)
	Total:	

Snack:	Amount	Calories (kcal)
	Total:	

Cups of Water: ☐☐☐☐☐☐☐☐ **Servings of Fruits/Veggies:** ☐☐☐☐☐☐☐☐

Exercise:	Duration	Calories (kcal) burned

DATE: Su Mo Tu We Th Fr Sa

Breakfast:	Amount	Calories (kcal)
	Total:	

Snack:	Amount	Calories (kcal)
	Total:	

Lunch:	Amount	Calories (kcal)
	Total:	

Snack:	Amount	Calories (kcal)
	Total:	

Dinner:	Amount	Calories (kcal)
	Total:	

Snack:	Amount	Calories (kcal)
	Total:	

Cups of Water: □□□□□□□□ **Servings of Fruits/Veggies:** □□□□□□□□

Exercise:	Duration	Calories (kcal) burned

DATE: Su Mo Tu We Th Fr Sa

Breakfast:	Amount	Calories (kcal)
	Total:	

Snack:	Amount	Calories (kcal)
	Total:	

Lunch:	Amount	Calories (kcal)
	Total:	

Snack:	Amount	Calories (kcal)
	Total:	
Dinner:	Amount	Calories (kcal)
	Total:	
Snack:	Amount	Calories (kcal)
	Total:	

Cups of Water: ☐☐☐☐☐☐☐☐ **Servings of Fruits/Veggies:** ☐☐☐☐☐☐☐☐

Exercise:	Duration	Calories (kcal) burned

DATE: Su Mo Tu We Th Fr Sa

Breakfast:	Amount	Calories (kcal)
	Total:	
Snack:	Amount	Calories (kcal)
	Total:	
Lunch:	Amount	Calories (kcal)
	Total:	

Snack:	Amount	Calories (kcal)
	Total:	
Dinner:	Amount	Calories (kcal)
	Total:	
Snack:	Amount	Calories (kcal)
	Total:	

Cups of Water: ☐☐☐☐☐☐☐☐ **Servings of Fruits/Veggies:** ☐☐☐☐☐☐☐☐

Exercise:	Duration	Calories (kcal) burned

DATE: **Su Mo Tu We Th Fr Sa**

Breakfast:	Amount	Calories (kcal)
	Total:	
Snack:	Amount	Calories (kcal)
	Total:	
Lunch:	Amount	Calories (kcal)
	Total:	

Snack:	Amount	Calories (kcal)
	Total:	
Dinner:	Amount	Calories (kcal)
	Total:	
Snack:	Amount	Calories (kcal)
	Total:	

Cups of Water: □□□□□□□□ **Servings of Fruits/Veggies:** □□□□□□□□

Exercise:	Duration	Calories (kcal) burned

DATE: Su Mo Tu We Th Fr Sa

Breakfast:	Amount	Calories (kcal)
	Total:	

Snack:	Amount	Calories (kcal)
	Total:	

Lunch:	Amount	Calories (kcal)
	Total:	

Snack:	Amount	Calories (kcal)
	Total:	
Dinner:	Amount	Calories (kcal)
	Total:	
Snack:	Amount	Calories (kcal)
	Total:	

Cups of Water: ☐☐☐☐☐☐☐☐☐☐ **Servings of Fruits/Veggies:** ☐☐☐☐☐☐☐☐☐☐

Exercise:	Duration	Calories (kcal) burned

DATE: Su Mo Tu We Th Fr Sa

Breakfast:	Amount	Calories (kcal)
	Total:	
Snack:	Amount	Calories (kcal)
	Total:	
Lunch:	Amount	Calories (kcal)
	Total:	

Snack:	Amount	Calories (kcal)
	Total:	
Dinner:	Amount	Calories (kcal)
	Total:	
Snack:	Amount	Calories (kcal)
	Total:	
Cups of Water: □□□□□□□□ **Servings of Fruits/Veggies:** □□□□□□□□		
Exercise:	Duration	Calories (kcal) burned

DATE: Su Mo Tu We Th Fr Sa

Breakfast:	Amount	Calories (kcal)
	Total:	
Snack:	Amount	Calories (kcal)
	Total:	
Lunch:	Amount	Calories (kcal)
	Total:	

Snack:	Amount	Calories (kcal)
	Total:	
Dinner:	Amount	Calories (kcal)
	Total:	
Snack:	Amount	Calories (kcal)
	Total:	

Cups of Water: □□□□□□□□ **Servings of Fruits/Veggies:** □□□□□□□□

Exercise:	Duration	Calories (kcal) burned

DATE: Su Mo Tu We Th Fr Sa

Breakfast:	Amount	Calories (kcal)
	Total:	
Snack:	Amount	Calories (kcal)
	Total:	
Lunch:	Amount	Calories (kcal)
	Total:	

Snack:	Amount	Calories (kcal)
	Total:	
Dinner:	Amount	Calories (kcal)
	Total:	
Snack:	Amount	Calories (kcal)
	Total:	

Cups of Water: □□□□□□□□ **Servings of Fruits/Veggies:** □□□□□□□□

Exercise:	Duration	Calories (kcal) burned

DATE: Su Mo Tu We Th Fr Sa

Breakfast:	Amount	Calories (kcal)
	Total:	
Snack:	Amount	Calories (kcal)
	Total:	
Lunch:	Amount	Calories (kcal)
	Total:	

Snack:	Amount	Calories (kcal)
	Total:	

Dinner:	Amount	Calories (kcal)
	Total:	

Snack:	Amount	Calories (kcal)
	Total:	

Cups of Water: □□□□□□□□ **Servings of Fruits/Veggies:** □□□□□□□□

Exercise:	Duration	Calories (kcal) burned

DATE: Su Mo Tu We Th Fr Sa

Breakfast:	Amount	Calories (kcal)
	Total:	

Snack:	Amount	Calories (kcal)
	Total:	

Lunch:	Amount	Calories (kcal)
	Total:	

Snack:	Amount	Calories (kcal)
	Total:	
Dinner:	Amount	Calories (kcal)
	Total:	
Snack:	Amount	Calories (kcal)
	Total:	

Cups of Water: □□□□□□□□ **Servings of Fruits/Veggies:** □□□□□□□□

Exercise:	Duration	Calories (kcal) burned

DATE: Su Mo Tu We Th Fr Sa

Breakfast:	Amount	Calories (kcal)
	Total:	
Snack:	Amount	Calories (kcal)
	Total:	
Lunch:	Amount	Calories (kcal)
	Total:	

Snack:	Amount	Calories (kcal)
	Total:	

Dinner:	Amount	Calories (kcal)
	Total:	

Snack:	Amount	Calories (kcal)
	Total:	

Cups of Water: ☐☐☐☐☐☐☐☐ **Servings of Fruits/Veggies:** ☐☐☐☐☐☐☐☐

Exercise:	Duration	Calories (kcal) burned

DATE: Su Mo Tu We Th Fr Sa

Breakfast:	Amount	Calories (kcal)
	Total:	

Snack:	Amount	Calories (kcal)
	Total:	

Lunch:	Amount	Calories (kcal)
	Total:	

Snack:	Amount	Calories (kcal)
	Total:	

Dinner:	Amount	Calories (kcal)
	Total:	

Snack:	Amount	Calories (kcal)
	Total:	

Cups of Water: ☐☐☐☐☐☐☐☐☐ Servings of Fruits/Veggies: ☐☐☐☐☐☐☐☐☐

Exercise:	Duration	Calories (kcal) burned

DATE: Su Mo Tu We Th Fr Sa

Breakfast:	Amount	Calories (kcal)
	Total:	
Snack:	Amount	Calories (kcal)
	Total:	
Lunch:	Amount	Calories (kcal)
	Total:	

Snack:	Amount	Calories (kcal)
	Total:	

Dinner:	Amount	Calories (kcal)
	Total:	

Snack:	Amount	Calories (kcal)
	Total:	

Cups of Water: ☐☐☐☐☐☐☐☐ **Servings of Fruits/Veggies:** ☐☐☐☐☐☐☐☐

Exercise:	Duration	Calories (kcal) burned

DATE: Su Mo Tu We Th Fr Sa

Breakfast:	Amount	Calories (kcal)
	Total:	

Snack:	Amount	Calories (kcal)
	Total:	

Lunch:	Amount	Calories (kcal)
	Total:	

Snack:	Amount	Calories (kcal)
	Total:	

Dinner:	Amount	Calories (kcal)
	Total:	

Snack:	Amount	Calories (kcal)
	Total:	

Cups of Water: □□□□□□□□ **Servings of Fruits/Veggies:** □□□□□□□□

Exercise:	Duration	Calories (kcal) burned

DATE: Su Mo Tu We Th Fr Sa

Breakfast:	Amount	Calories (kcal)
	Total:	

Snack:	Amount	Calories (kcal)
	Total:	

Lunch:	Amount	Calories (kcal)
	Total:	

Snack:	Amount	Calories (kcal)
	Total:	

Dinner:	Amount	Calories (kcal)
	Total:	

Snack:	Amount	Calories (kcal)
	Total:	

Cups of Water: □□□□□□□□□ **Servings of Fruits/Veggies:** □□□□□□□□□

Exercise:	Duration	Calories (kcal) burned

DATE: Su Mo Tu We Th Fr Sa

Breakfast:	Amount	Calories (kcal)
	Total:	

Snack:	Amount	Calories (kcal)
	Total:	

Lunch:	Amount	Calories (kcal)
	Total:	

Snack:	Amount	Calories (kcal)
	Total:	

Dinner:	Amount	Calories (kcal)
	Total:	

Snack:	Amount	Calories (kcal)
	Total:	

Cups of Water: ☐☐☐☐☐☐☐☐☐ **Servings of Fruits/Veggies:** ☐☐☐☐☐☐☐☐☐

Exercise:	Duration	Calories (kcal) burned

DATE: Su Mo Tu We Th Fr Sa

Breakfast:	Amount	Calories (kcal)
	Total:	
Snack:	Amount	Calories (kcal)
	Total:	
Lunch:	Amount	Calories (kcal)
	Total:	

Snack:	Amount	Calories (kcal)
	Total:	

Dinner:	Amount	Calories (kcal)
	Total:	

Snack:	Amount	Calories (kcal)
	Total:	

Cups of Water: □□□□□□□□ **Servings of Fruits/Veggies:** □□□□□□□□

Exercise:	Duration	Calories (kcal) burned

DATE: Su Mo Tu We Th Fr Sa

Breakfast:	Amount	Calories (kcal)
	Total:	

Snack:	Amount	Calories (kcal)
	Total:	

Lunch:	Amount	Calories (kcal)
	Total:	

Snack:	Amount	Calories (kcal)
	Total:	

Dinner:	Amount	Calories (kcal)
	Total:	

Snack:	Amount	Calories (kcal)
	Total:	

Cups of Water: □□□□□□□□ **Servings of Fruits/Veggies:** □□□□□□□□

Exercise:	Duration	Calories (kcal) burned

DATE: Su Mo Tu We Th Fr Sa

Breakfast:	Amount	Calories (kcal)
	Total:	

Snack:	Amount	Calories (kcal)
	Total:	

Lunch:	Amount	Calories (kcal)
	Total:	

Snack:	Amount	Calories (kcal)
	Total:	

Dinner:	Amount	Calories (kcal)
	Total:	

Snack:	Amount	Calories (kcal)
	Total:	

Cups of Water: ☐☐☐☐☐☐☐☐ **Servings of Fruits/Veggies:** ☐☐☐☐☐☐☐☐

Exercise:	Duration	Calories (kcal) burned

DATE: Su Mo Tu We Th Fr Sa

Breakfast:	Amount	Calories (kcal)
	Total:	
Snack:	Amount	Calories (kcal)
	Total:	
Lunch:	Amount	Calories (kcal)
	Total:	

Snack:	Amount	Calories (kcal)
	Total:	
Dinner:	Amount	Calories (kcal)
	Total:	
Snack:	Amount	Calories (kcal)
	Total:	

Cups of Water: ☐☐☐☐☐☐☐☐ **Servings of Fruits/Veggies:** ☐☐☐☐☐☐☐☐

Exercise:	Duration	Calories (kcal) burned

DATE: Su Mo Tu We Th Fr Sa

Breakfast:	Amount	Calories (kcal)
	Total:	
Snack:	Amount	Calories (kcal)
	Total:	
Lunch:	Amount	Calories (kcal)
	Total:	

Snack:	Amount	Calories (kcal)
	Total:	

Dinner:	Amount	Calories (kcal)
	Total:	

Snack:	Amount	Calories (kcal)
	Total:	

Cups of Water: □□□□□□□□ Servings of Fruits/Veggies: □□□□□□□□

Exercise:	Duration	Calories (kcal) burned

DATE: Su Mo Tu We Th Fr Sa

Breakfast:	Amount	Calories (kcal)
	Total:	
Snack:	Amount	Calories (kcal)
	Total:	
Lunch:	Amount	Calories (kcal)
	Total:	

Snack:	Amount	Calories (kcal)
	Total:	
Dinner:	Amount	Calories (kcal)
	Total:	
Snack:	Amount	Calories (kcal)
	Total:	
Cups of Water: □□□□□□□□ **Servings of Fruits/Veggies:** □□□□□□□□		
Exercise:	Duration	Calories (kcal) burned

DATE: **Su Mo Tu We Th Fr Sa**

Breakfast:	Amount	Calories (kcal)
	Total:	
Snack:	Amount	Calories (kcal)
	Total:	
Lunch:	Amount	Calories (kcal)
	Total:	

Snack:	Amount	Calories (kcal)
	Total:	

Dinner:	Amount	Calories (kcal)
	Total:	

Snack:	Amount	Calories (kcal)
	Total:	

Cups of Water: □□□□□□□□ Servings of Fruits/Veggies: □□□□□□□□

Exercise:	Duration	Calories (kcal) burned

DATE: Su Mo Tu We Th Fr Sa

Breakfast:	Amount	Calories (kcal)
	Total:	
Snack:	Amount	Calories (kcal)
	Total:	
Lunch:	Amount	Calories (kcal)
	Total:	

Snack:	Amount	Calories (kcal)
	Total:	
Dinner:	Amount	Calories (kcal)
	Total:	
Snack:	Amount	Calories (kcal)
	Total:	
Cups of Water: □□□□□□□□ **Servings of Fruits/Veggies:** □□□□□□□□		
Exercise:	Duration	Calories (kcal) burned

DATE: Su Mo Tu We Th Fr Sa

Breakfast:	Amount	Calories (kcal)
	Total:	

Snack:	Amount	Calories (kcal)
	Total:	

Lunch:	Amount	Calories (kcal)
	Total:	

Snack:	Amount	Calories (kcal)
	Total:	

Dinner:	Amount	Calories (kcal)
	Total:	

Snack:	Amount	Calories (kcal)
	Total:	

Cups of Water: □□□□□□□□ **Servings of Fruits/Veggies:** □□□□□□□□

Exercise:	Duration	Calories (kcal) burned

DATE: Su Mo Tu We Th Fr Sa

Breakfast:	Amount	Calories (kcal)
	Total:	
Snack:	Amount	Calories (kcal)
	Total:	
Lunch:	Amount	Calories (kcal)
	Total:	

Snack:	Amount	Calories (kcal)
	Total:	

Dinner:	Amount	Calories (kcal)
	Total:	

Snack:	Amount	Calories (kcal)
	Total:	

Cups of Water: □□□□□□□□ **Servings of Fruits/Veggies:** □□□□□□□□

Exercise:	Duration	Calories (kcal) burned

DATE: Su Mo Tu We Th Fr Sa

Breakfast:	Amount	Calories (kcal)
	Total:	

Snack:	Amount	Calories (kcal)
	Total:	

Lunch:	Amount	Calories (kcal)
	Total:	

Snack:	Amount	Calories (kcal)
	Total:	
Dinner:	Amount	Calories (kcal)
	Total:	
Snack:	Amount	Calories (kcal)
	Total:	
Cups of Water: □□□□□□□□ **Servings of Fruits/Veggies:** □□□□□□□□		
Exercise:	Duration	Calories (kcal) burned

DATE: Su Mo Tu We Th Fr Sa

Breakfast:	Amount	Calories (kcal)
	Total:	
Snack:	Amount	Calories (kcal)
	Total:	
Lunch:	Amount	Calories (kcal)
	Total:	

Snack:	Amount	Calories (kcal)
	Total:	

Dinner:	Amount	Calories (kcal)
	Total:	

Snack:	Amount	Calories (kcal)
	Total:	

Cups of Water: ☐☐☐☐☐☐☐☐ **Servings of Fruits/Veggies:** ☐☐☐☐☐☐☐☐

Exercise:	Duration	Calories (kcal) burned

DATE: Su Mo Tu We Th Fr Sa

Breakfast:	Amount	Calories (kcal)
	Total:	

Snack:	Amount	Calories (kcal)
	Total:	

Lunch:	Amount	Calories (kcal)
	Total:	

Snack:	Amount	Calories (kcal)
	Total:	

Dinner:	Amount	Calories (kcal)
	Total:	

Snack:	Amount	Calories (kcal)
	Total:	

Cups of Water: □□□□□□□□ **Servings of Fruits/Veggies:** □□□□□□□□

Exercise:	Duration	Calories (kcal) burned

DATE: Su Mo Tu We Th Fr Sa

Breakfast:	Amount	Calories (kcal)
	Total:	
Snack:	Amount	Calories (kcal)
	Total:	
Lunch:	Amount	Calories (kcal)
	Total:	

Snack:	Amount	Calories (kcal)
	Total:	

Dinner:	Amount	Calories (kcal)
	Total:	

Snack:	Amount	Calories (kcal)
	Total:	

Cups of Water: □□□□□□□□ **Servings of Fruits/Veggies:** □□□□□□□□

Exercise:	Duration	Calories (kcal) burned

DATE: Su Mo Tu We Th Fr Sa

Breakfast:	Amount	Calories (kcal)
	Total:	

Snack:	Amount	Calories (kcal)
	Total:	

Lunch:	Amount	Calories (kcal)
	Total:	

Snack:	Amount	Calories (kcal)
	Total:	

Dinner:	Amount	Calories (kcal)
	Total:	

Snack:	Amount	Calories (kcal)
	Total:	

Cups of Water: □□□□□□□□ **Servings of Fruits/Veggies:** □□□□□□□□

Exercise:	Duration	Calories (kcal) burned

DATE: Su Mo Tu We Th Fr Sa

Breakfast:	Amount	Calories (kcal)
	Total:	
Snack:	Amount	Calories (kcal)
	Total:	
Lunch:	Amount	Calories (kcal)
	Total:	

Snack:	Amount	Calories (kcal)
	Total:	

Dinner:	Amount	Calories (kcal)
	Total:	

Snack:	Amount	Calories (kcal)
	Total:	

Cups of Water: □□□□□□□□ **Servings of Fruits/Veggies:** □□□□□□□□

Exercise:	Duration	Calories (kcal) burned

DATE: Su Mo Tu We Th Fr Sa

Breakfast:	Amount	Calories (kcal)
	Total:	
Snack:	Amount	Calories (kcal)
	Total:	
Lunch:	Amount	Calories (kcal)
	Total:	

Snack:	Amount	Calories (kcal)
	Total:	

Dinner:	Amount	Calories (kcal)
	Total:	

Snack:	Amount	Calories (kcal)
	Total:	

Cups of Water: ☐☐☐☐☐☐☐☐ Servings of Fruits/Veggies: ☐☐☐☐☐☐☐☐

Exercise:	Duration	Calories (kcal) burned

DATE: Su Mo Tu We Th Fr Sa

Breakfast:	Amount	Calories (kcal)
	Total:	
Snack:	Amount	Calories (kcal)
	Total:	
Lunch:	Amount	Calories (kcal)
	Total:	

Snack:	Amount	Calories (kcal)
	Total:	
Dinner:	Amount	Calories (kcal)
	Total:	
Snack:	Amount	Calories (kcal)
	Total:	

Cups of Water: □□□□□□□□ **Servings of Fruits/Veggies:** □□□□□□□□

Exercise:	Duration	Calories (kcal) burned

DATE: Su Mo Tu We Th Fr Sa

Breakfast:	Amount	Calories (kcal)
	Total:	
Snack:	Amount	Calories (kcal)
	Total:	
Lunch:	Amount	Calories (kcal)
	Total:	

Snack:	Amount	Calories (kcal)
	Total:	

Dinner:	Amount	Calories (kcal)
	Total:	

Snack:	Amount	Calories (kcal)
	Total:	

Cups of Water: ☐☐☐☐☐☐☐☐☐ Servings of Fruits/Veggies: ☐☐☐☐☐☐☐☐☐

Exercise:	Duration	Calories (kcal) burned

DATE: Su Mo Tu We Th Fr Sa

Breakfast:	Amount	Calories (kcal)
	Total:	
Snack:	Amount	Calories (kcal)
	Total:	
Lunch:	Amount	Calories (kcal)
	Total:	

Snack:	Amount	Calories (kcal)
	Total:	

Dinner:	Amount	Calories (kcal)
	Total:	

Snack:	Amount	Calories (kcal)
	Total:	

Cups of Water: □□□□□□□□ **Servings of Fruits/Veggies:** □□□□□□□□

Exercise:	Duration	Calories (kcal) burned

DATE: Su Mo Tu We Th Fr Sa

Breakfast:	Amount	Calories (kcal)
	Total:	

Snack:	Amount	Calories (kcal)
	Total:	

Lunch:	Amount	Calories (kcal)
	Total:	

Snack:	Amount	Calories (kcal)
	Total:	

Dinner:	Amount	Calories (kcal)
	Total:	

Snack:	Amount	Calories (kcal)
	Total:	

Cups of Water: ☐☐☐☐☐☐☐☐ **Servings of Fruits/Veggies:** ☐☐☐☐☐☐☐☐

Exercise:	Duration	Calories (kcal) burned

DATE: Su Mo Tu We Th Fr Sa

Breakfast:	Amount	Calories (kcal)
	Total:	

Snack:	Amount	Calories (kcal)
	Total:	

Lunch:	Amount	Calories (kcal)
	Total:	

Snack:	Amount	Calories (kcal)
	Total:	
Dinner:	Amount	Calories (kcal)
	Total:	
Snack:	Amount	Calories (kcal)
	Total:	

Cups of Water: ☐☐☐☐☐☐☐☐ **Servings of Fruits/Veggies:** ☐☐☐☐☐☐☐☐

Exercise:	Duration	Calories (kcal) burned

DATE: Su Mo Tu We Th Fr Sa

Breakfast:	Amount	Calories (kcal)
	Total:	
Snack:	Amount	Calories (kcal)
	Total:	
Lunch:	Amount	Calories (kcal)
	Total:	

Snack:	Amount	Calories (kcal)
	Total:	

Dinner:	Amount	Calories (kcal)
	Total:	

Snack:	Amount	Calories (kcal)
	Total:	

Cups of Water: □□□□□□□□ **Servings of Fruits/Veggies:** □□□□□□□□

Exercise:	Duration	Calories (kcal) burned

DATE: Su Mo Tu We Th Fr Sa

Breakfast:	Amount	Calories (kcal)
	Total:	

Snack:	Amount	Calories (kcal)
	Total:	

Lunch:	Amount	Calories (kcal)
	Total:	

Snack:	Amount	Calories (kcal)
	Total:	

Dinner:	Amount	Calories (kcal)
	Total:	

Snack:	Amount	Calories (kcal)
	Total:	

Cups of Water: □□□□□□□□□ **Servings of Fruits/Veggies:** □□□□□□□□□

Exercise:	Duration	Calories (kcal) burned

DATE: Su Mo Tu We Th Fr Sa

Breakfast:	Amount	Calories (kcal)
	Total:	

Snack:	Amount	Calories (kcal)
	Total:	

Lunch:	Amount	Calories (kcal)
	Total:	

Snack:	Amount	Calories (kcal)
	Total:	

Dinner:	Amount	Calories (kcal)
	Total:	

Snack:	Amount	Calories (kcal)
	Total:	

Cups of Water: □□□□□□□□ **Servings of Fruits/Veggies:** □□□□□□□□

Exercise:	Duration	Calories (kcal) burned

DATE: Su Mo Tu We Th Fr Sa

Breakfast:	Amount	Calories (kcal)
	Total:	

Snack:	Amount	Calories (kcal)
	Total:	

Lunch:	Amount	Calories (kcal)
	Total:	

Snack:	Amount	Calories (kcal)
	Total:	

Dinner:	Amount	Calories (kcal)
	Total:	

Snack:	Amount	Calories (kcal)
	Total:	

Cups of Water: □□□□□□□□□ **Servings of Fruits/Veggies:** □□□□□□□□□

Exercise:	Duration	Calories (kcal) burned

DATE: Su Mo Tu We Th Fr Sa

Breakfast:	Amount	Calories (kcal)
	Total:	
Snack:	Amount	Calories (kcal)
	Total:	
Lunch:	Amount	Calories (kcal)
	Total:	

Snack:	Amount	Calories (kcal)
	Total:	

Dinner:	Amount	Calories (kcal)
	Total:	

Snack:	Amount	Calories (kcal)
	Total:	

Cups of Water: □□□□□□□□ **Servings of Fruits/Veggies:** □□□□□□□□

Exercise:	Duration	Calories (kcal) burned

DATE: Su Mo Tu We Th Fr Sa

Breakfast:	Amount	Calories (kcal)
	Total:	

Snack:	Amount	Calories (kcal)
	Total:	

Lunch:	Amount	Calories (kcal)
	Total:	

Snack:	Amount	Calories (kcal)
	Total:	

Dinner:	Amount	Calories (kcal)
	Total:	

Snack:	Amount	Calories (kcal)
	Total:	

Cups of Water: □□□□□□□□ **Servings of Fruits/Veggies:** □□□□□□□□

Exercise:	Duration	Calories (kcal) burned

DATE: Su Mo Tu We Th Fr Sa

Breakfast:	Amount	Calories (kcal)
	Total:	

Snack:	Amount	Calories (kcal)
	Total:	

Lunch:	Amount	Calories (kcal)
	Total:	

Snack:	Amount	Calories (kcal)
	Total:	

Dinner:	Amount	Calories (kcal)
	Total:	

Snack:	Amount	Calories (kcal)
	Total:	

Cups of Water: □□□□□□□□ **Servings of Fruits/Veggies:** □□□□□□□□

Exercise:	Duration	Calories (kcal) burned

DATE: Su Mo Tu We Th Fr Sa

Breakfast:	Amount	Calories (kcal)
	Total:	
Snack:	Amount	Calories (kcal)
	Total:	
Lunch:	Amount	Calories (kcal)
	Total:	

Snack:	Amount	Calories (kcal)
	Total:	

Dinner:	Amount	Calories (kcal)
	Total:	

Snack:	Amount	Calories (kcal)
	Total:	

Cups of Water: ☐☐☐☐☐☐☐☐ **Servings of Fruits/Veggies:** ☐☐☐☐☐☐☐☐

Exercise:	Duration	Calories (kcal) burned

DATE: **Su Mo Tu We Th Fr Sa**

Breakfast:	Amount	Calories (kcal)
	Total:	
Snack:	Amount	Calories (kcal)
	Total:	
Lunch:	Amount	Calories (kcal)
	Total:	

Snack:	Amount	Calories (kcal)
	Total:	
Dinner:	Amount	Calories (kcal)
	Total:	
Snack:	Amount	Calories (kcal)
	Total:	
Cups of Water: □□□□□□□□ **Servings of Fruits/Veggies:** □□□□□□□□		
Exercise:	Duration	Calories (kcal) burned

DATE: Su Mo Tu We Th Fr Sa

Breakfast:	Amount	Calories (kcal)
	Total:	
Snack:	Amount	Calories (kcal)
	Total:	
Lunch:	Amount	Calories (kcal)
	Total:	

Snack:	Amount	Calories (kcal)
	Total:	

Dinner:	Amount	Calories (kcal)
	Total:	

Snack:	Amount	Calories (kcal)
	Total:	

Cups of Water: □□□□□□□□ **Servings of Fruits/Veggies:** □□□□□□□□

Exercise:	Duration	Calories (kcal) burned

DATE: Su Mo Tu We Th Fr Sa

Breakfast:	Amount	Calories (kcal)
	Total:	
Snack:	Amount	Calories (kcal)
	Total:	
Lunch:	Amount	Calories (kcal)
	Total:	

Snack:	Amount	Calories (kcal)
	Total:	

Dinner:	Amount	Calories (kcal)
	Total:	

Snack:	Amount	Calories (kcal)
	Total:	

Cups of Water: ☐☐☐☐☐☐☐☐ Servings of Fruits/Veggies: ☐☐☐☐☐☐☐☐

Exercise:	Duration	Calories (kcal) burned

DATE: Su Mo Tu We Th Fr Sa

Breakfast:	Amount	Calories (kcal)
	Total:	
Snack:	Amount	Calories (kcal)
	Total:	
Lunch:	Amount	Calories (kcal)
	Total:	

Snack:	Amount	Calories (kcal)
	Total:	

Dinner:	Amount	Calories (kcal)
	Total:	

Snack:	Amount	Calories (kcal)
	Total:	

Cups of Water: □□□□□□□□ Servings of Fruits/Veggies: □□□□□□□□

Exercise:	Duration	Calories (kcal) burned

DATE: Su Mo Tu We Th Fr Sa

Breakfast:	Amount	Calories (kcal)
	Total:	

Snack:	Amount	Calories (kcal)
	Total:	

Lunch:	Amount	Calories (kcal)
	Total:	

Snack:	Amount	Calories (kcal)
	Total:	

Dinner:	Amount	Calories (kcal)
	Total:	

Snack:	Amount	Calories (kcal)
	Total:	

Cups of Water: □□□□□□□□ **Servings of Fruits/Veggies:** □□□□□□□□

Exercise:	Duration	Calories (kcal) burned

DATE: Su Mo Tu We Th Fr Sa

Breakfast:	Amount	Calories (kcal)
	Total:	

Snack:	Amount	Calories (kcal)
	Total:	

Lunch:	Amount	Calories (kcal)
	Total:	

Snack:	Amount	Calories (kcal)
	Total:	
Dinner:	Amount	Calories (kcal)
	Total:	
Snack:	Amount	Calories (kcal)
	Total:	

Cups of Water: □□□□□□□□ **Servings of Fruits/Veggies:** □□□□□□□□

Exercise:	Duration	Calories (kcal) burned

DATE: Su Mo Tu We Th Fr Sa

Breakfast:	Amount	Calories (kcal)
	Total:	
Snack:	Amount	Calories (kcal)
	Total:	
Lunch:	Amount	Calories (kcal)
	Total:	

Snack:	Amount	Calories (kcal)
	Total:	

Dinner:	Amount	Calories (kcal)
	Total:	

Snack:	Amount	Calories (kcal)
	Total:	

Cups of Water: ☐☐☐☐☐☐☐☐ **Servings of Fruits/Veggies:** ☐☐☐☐☐☐☐☐

Exercise:	Duration	Calories (kcal) burned

DATE: **Su Mo Tu We Th Fr Sa**

Breakfast:	Amount	Calories (kcal)
	Total:	
Snack:	Amount	Calories (kcal)
	Total:	
Lunch:	Amount	Calories (kcal)
	Total:	

Snack:	Amount	Calories (kcal)
	Total:	

Dinner:	Amount	Calories (kcal)
	Total:	

Snack:	Amount	Calories (kcal)
	Total:	

Cups of Water: □□□□□□□□ **Servings of Fruits/Veggies:** □□□□□□□□

Exercise:	Duration	Calories (kcal) burned

DATE: Su Mo Tu We Th Fr Sa

Breakfast:	Amount	Calories (kcal)
	Total:	

Snack:	Amount	Calories (kcal)
	Total:	

Lunch:	Amount	Calories (kcal)
	Total:	

Snack:	Amount	Calories (kcal)
	Total:	

Dinner:	Amount	Calories (kcal)
	Total:	

Snack:	Amount	Calories (kcal)
	Total:	

Cups of Water: ☐☐☐☐☐☐☐☐ **Servings of Fruits/Veggies:** ☐☐☐☐☐☐☐☐

Exercise:	Duration	Calories (kcal) burned

DATE: Su Mo Tu We Th Fr Sa

Breakfast:	Amount	Calories (kcal)
	Total:	

Snack:	Amount	Calories (kcal)
	Total:	

Lunch:	Amount	Calories (kcal)
	Total:	

Snack:	Amount	Calories (kcal)
	Total:	

Dinner:	Amount	Calories (kcal)
	Total:	

Snack:	Amount	Calories (kcal)
	Total:	

Cups of Water: □□□□□□□□ **Servings of Fruits/Veggies:** □□□□□□□□

Exercise:	Duration	Calories (kcal) burned

DATE: Su Mo Tu We Th Fr Sa

Breakfast:	Amount	Calories (kcal)
	Total:	
Snack:	Amount	Calories (kcal)
	Total:	
Lunch:	Amount	Calories (kcal)
	Total:	

Snack:	Amount	Calories (kcal)
	Total:	

Dinner:	Amount	Calories (kcal)
	Total:	

Snack:	Amount	Calories (kcal)
	Total:	

Cups of Water: ☐☐☐☐☐☐☐☐ **Servings of Fruits/Veggies:** ☐☐☐☐☐☐☐☐

Exercise:	Duration	Calories (kcal) burned

DATE: Su Mo Tu We Th Fr Sa

Breakfast:	Amount	Calories (kcal)
	Total:	
Snack:	Amount	Calories (kcal)
	Total:	
Lunch:	Amount	Calories (kcal)
	Total:	

Snack:	Amount	Calories (kcal)
	Total:	

Dinner:	Amount	Calories (kcal)
	Total:	

Snack:	Amount	Calories (kcal)
	Total:	

Cups of Water: ☐☐☐☐☐☐☐☐ **Servings of Fruits/Veggies:** ☐☐☐☐☐☐☐☐

Exercise:	Duration	Calories (kcal) burned

DATE: Su Mo Tu We Th Fr Sa

Breakfast:	Amount	Calories (kcal)
	Total:	

Snack:	Amount	Calories (kcal)
	Total:	

Lunch:	Amount	Calories (kcal)
	Total:	

Snack:	Amount	Calories (kcal)
	Total:	
Dinner:	Amount	Calories (kcal)
	Total:	
Snack:	Amount	Calories (kcal)
	Total:	

Cups of Water: □□□□□□□□ **Servings of Fruits/Veggies:** □□□□□□□□

Exercise:	Duration	Calories (kcal) burned

DATE: Su Mo Tu We Th Fr Sa

Breakfast:	Amount	Calories (kcal)
	Total:	
Snack:	Amount	Calories (kcal)
	Total:	
Lunch:	Amount	Calories (kcal)
	Total:	

Snack:	Amount	Calories (kcal)
	Total:	

Dinner:	Amount	Calories (kcal)
	Total:	

Snack:	Amount	Calories (kcal)
	Total:	

Cups of Water: □□□□□□□□ Servings of Fruits/Veggies: □□□□□□□□

Exercise:	Duration	Calories (kcal) burned

DATE: Su Mo Tu We Th Fr Sa

Breakfast:	Amount	Calories (kcal)
	Total:	
Snack:	Amount	Calories (kcal)
	Total:	
Lunch:	Amount	Calories (kcal)
	Total:	

Snack:	Amount	Calories (kcal)
	Total:	

Dinner:	Amount	Calories (kcal)
	Total:	

Snack:	Amount	Calories (kcal)
	Total:	

Cups of Water: ☐☐☐☐☐☐☐☐ **Servings of Fruits/Veggies:** ☐☐☐☐☐☐☐☐

Exercise:	Duration	Calories (kcal) burned

DATE: Su Mo Tu We Th Fr Sa

Breakfast:	Amount	Calories (kcal)
	Total:	

Snack:	Amount	Calories (kcal)
	Total:	

Lunch:	Amount	Calories (kcal)
	Total:	

Snack:	Amount	Calories (kcal)
	Total:	
Dinner:	Amount	Calories (kcal)
	Total:	
Snack:	Amount	Calories (kcal)
	Total:	

Cups of Water: ☐☐☐☐☐☐☐☐ **Servings of Fruits/Veggies:** ☐☐☐☐☐☐☐☐

Exercise:	Duration	Calories (kcal) burned

DATE: **Su Mo Tu We Th Fr Sa**

Breakfast:	Amount	Calories (kcal)
	Total:	
Snack:	Amount	Calories (kcal)
	Total:	
Lunch:	Amount	Calories (kcal)
	Total:	

Snack:	Amount	Calories (kcal)
	Total:	

Dinner:	Amount	Calories (kcal)
	Total:	

Snack:	Amount	Calories (kcal)
	Total:	

Cups of Water: □□□□□□□□ **Servings of Fruits/Veggies:** □□□□□□□□

Exercise:	Duration	Calories (kcal) burned

DATE: Su Mo Tu We Th Fr Sa

Breakfast:	Amount	Calories (kcal)
	Total:	

Snack:	Amount	Calories (kcal)
	Total:	

Lunch:	Amount	Calories (kcal)
	Total:	

Snack:	Amount	Calories (kcal)
	Total:	

Dinner:	Amount	Calories (kcal)
	Total:	

Snack:	Amount	Calories (kcal)
	Total:	

Cups of Water: □□□□□□□□ **Servings of Fruits/Veggies:** □□□□□□□□

Exercise:	Duration	Calories (kcal) burned

DATE: Su Mo Tu We Th Fr Sa

Breakfast:	Amount	Calories (kcal)
	Total:	

Snack:	Amount	Calories (kcal)
	Total:	

Lunch:	Amount	Calories (kcal)
	Total:	

Snack:	Amount	Calories (kcal)
	Total:	

Dinner:	Amount	Calories (kcal)
	Total:	

Snack:	Amount	Calories (kcal)
	Total:	

Cups of Water: ☐☐☐☐☐☐☐☐ **Servings of Fruits/Veggies:** ☐☐☐☐☐☐☐☐

Exercise:	Duration	Calories (kcal) burned

DATE: Su Mo Tu We Th Fr Sa

Breakfast:	Amount	Calories (kcal)
	Total:	
Snack:	Amount	Calories (kcal)
	Total:	
Lunch:	Amount	Calories (kcal)
	Total:	

Snack:	Amount	Calories (kcal)
	Total:	

Dinner:	Amount	Calories (kcal)
	Total:	

Snack:	Amount	Calories (kcal)
	Total:	

Cups of Water: □□□□□□□□ Servings of Fruits/Veggies: □□□□□□□□

Exercise:	Duration	Calories (kcal) burned

DATE: Su Mo Tu We Th Fr Sa

Breakfast:	Amount	Calories (kcal)
	Total:	

Snack:	Amount	Calories (kcal)
	Total:	

Lunch:	Amount	Calories (kcal)
	Total:	

Snack:	Amount	Calories (kcal)
	Total:	

Dinner:	Amount	Calories (kcal)
	Total:	

Snack:	Amount	Calories (kcal)
	Total:	

Cups of Water: ☐☐☐☐☐☐☐☐ **Servings of Fruits/Veggies:** ☐☐☐☐☐☐☐☐

Exercise:	Duration	Calories (kcal) burned

DATE: Su Mo Tu We Th Fr Sa

Breakfast:	Amount	Calories (kcal)
	Total:	
Snack:	Amount	Calories (kcal)
	Total:	
Lunch:	Amount	Calories (kcal)
	Total:	

Snack:	Amount	Calories (kcal)
	Total:	

Dinner:	Amount	Calories (kcal)
	Total:	

Snack:	Amount	Calories (kcal)
	Total:	

Cups of Water: □□□□□□□□ **Servings of Fruits/Veggies:** □□□□□□□□

Exercise:	Duration	Calories (kcal) burned

DATE: Su Mo Tu We Th Fr Sa

Breakfast:	Amount	Calories (kcal)
	Total:	
Snack:	Amount	Calories (kcal)
	Total:	
Lunch:	Amount	Calories (kcal)
	Total:	

Snack:	Amount	Calories (kcal)
	Total:	

Dinner:	Amount	Calories (kcal)
	Total:	

Snack:	Amount	Calories (kcal)
	Total:	

Cups of Water: □□□□□□□□ **Servings of Fruits/Veggies:** □□□□□□□□

Exercise:	Duration	Calories (kcal) burned

DATE: Su Mo Tu We Th Fr Sa

Breakfast:	Amount	Calories (kcal)
	Total:	

Snack:	Amount	Calories (kcal)
	Total:	

Lunch:	Amount	Calories (kcal)
	Total:	

Snack:	Amount	Calories (kcal)
	Total:	

Dinner:	Amount	Calories (kcal)
	Total:	

Snack:	Amount	Calories (kcal)
	Total:	

Cups of Water: ☐☐☐☐☐☐☐☐ **Servings of Fruits/Veggies:** ☐☐☐☐☐☐☐☐

Exercise:	Duration	Calories (kcal) burned

DATE: Su Mo Tu We Th Fr Sa

Breakfast:	Amount	Calories (kcal)
	Total:	

Snack:	Amount	Calories (kcal)
	Total:	

Lunch:	Amount	Calories (kcal)
	Total:	

Snack:	Amount	Calories (kcal)
	Total:	
Dinner:	Amount	Calories (kcal)
	Total:	
Snack:	Amount	Calories (kcal)
	Total:	

Cups of Water: □□□□□□□□ **Servings of Fruits/Veggies:** □□□□□□□□

Exercise:	Duration	Calories (kcal) burned

DATE: Su Mo Tu We Th Fr Sa

Breakfast:	Amount	Calories (kcal)
	Total:	

Snack:	Amount	Calories (kcal)
	Total:	

Lunch:	Amount	Calories (kcal)
	Total:	

Snack:	Amount	Calories (kcal)
	Total:	

Dinner:	Amount	Calories (kcal)
	Total:	

Snack:	Amount	Calories (kcal)
	Total:	

Cups of Water: ☐☐☐☐☐☐☐☐☐ **Servings of Fruits/Veggies:** ☐☐☐☐☐☐☐☐☐

Exercise:	Duration	Calories (kcal) burned

DATE: Su Mo Tu We Th Fr Sa

Breakfast:	Amount	Calories (kcal)
	Total:	
Snack:	Amount	Calories (kcal)
	Total:	
Lunch:	Amount	Calories (kcal)
	Total:	

Snack:	Amount	Calories (kcal)
	Total:	

Dinner:	Amount	Calories (kcal)
	Total:	

Snack:	Amount	Calories (kcal)
	Total:	

Cups of Water: □□□□□□□□ **Servings of Fruits/Veggies:** □□□□□□□□

Exercise:	Duration	Calories (kcal) burned

DATE: Su Mo Tu We Th Fr Sa

Breakfast:	Amount	Calories (kcal)
	Total:	

Snack:	Amount	Calories (kcal)
	Total:	

Lunch:	Amount	Calories (kcal)
	Total:	

Snack:	Amount	Calories (kcal)
	Total:	

Dinner:	Amount	Calories (kcal)
	Total:	

Snack:	Amount	Calories (kcal)
	Total:	

Cups of Water: □□□□□□□□□ **Servings of Fruits/Veggies:** □□□□□□□□□

Exercise:	Duration	Calories (kcal) burned

DATE: Su Mo Tu We Th Fr Sa

Breakfast:	Amount	Calories (kcal)
	Total:	

Snack:	Amount	Calories (kcal)
	Total:	

Lunch:	Amount	Calories (kcal)
	Total:	

Snack:	Amount	Calories (kcal)
	Total:	

Dinner:	Amount	Calories (kcal)
	Total:	

Snack:	Amount	Calories (kcal)
	Total:	

Cups of Water: □□□□□□□□ **Servings of Fruits/Veggies:** □□□□□□□□

Exercise:	Duration	Calories (kcal) burned

DATE: Su Mo Tu We Th Fr Sa

Breakfast:	Amount	Calories (kcal)
	Total:	

Snack:	Amount	Calories (kcal)
	Total:	

Lunch:	Amount	Calories (kcal)
	Total:	

Snack:	Amount	Calories (kcal)
	Total:	

Dinner:	Amount	Calories (kcal)
	Total:	

Snack:	Amount	Calories (kcal)
	Total:	

Cups of Water: □□□□□□□□ Servings of Fruits/Veggies: □□□□□□□□

Exercise:	Duration	Calories (kcal) burned

DATE: Su Mo Tu We Th Fr Sa

Breakfast:	Amount	Calories (kcal)
	Total:	
Snack:	Amount	Calories (kcal)
	Total:	
Lunch:	Amount	Calories (kcal)
	Total:	

Snack:	Amount	Calories (kcal)
	Total:	

Dinner:	Amount	Calories (kcal)
	Total:	

Snack:	Amount	Calories (kcal)
	Total:	

Cups of Water: □□□□□□□□ **Servings of Fruits/Veggies:** □□□□□□□□

Exercise:	Duration	Calories (kcal) burned

DATE: Su Mo Tu We Th Fr Sa

Breakfast:	Amount	Calories (kcal)
	Total:	
Snack:	Amount	Calories (kcal)
	Total:	
Lunch:	Amount	Calories (kcal)
	Total:	

Snack:	Amount	Calories (kcal)
	Total:	

Dinner:	Amount	Calories (kcal)
	Total:	

Snack:	Amount	Calories (kcal)
	Total:	

Cups of Water: □□□□□□□□ **Servings of Fruits/Veggies:** □□□□□□□□

Exercise:	Duration	Calories (kcal) burned

DATE: **Su Mo Tu We Th Fr Sa**

Breakfast:	Amount	Calories (kcal)
	Total:	
Snack:	Amount	Calories (kcal)
	Total:	
Lunch:	Amount	Calories (kcal)
	Total:	

Snack:	Amount	Calories (kcal)
	Total:	

Dinner:	Amount	Calories (kcal)
	Total:	

Snack:	Amount	Calories (kcal)
	Total:	

Cups of Water: ☐☐☐☐☐☐☐☐ **Servings of Fruits/Veggies:** ☐☐☐☐☐☐☐☐

Exercise:	Duration	Calories (kcal) burned

DATE: Su Mo Tu We Th Fr Sa

Breakfast:	Amount	Calories (kcal)
	Total:	
Snack:	Amount	Calories (kcal)
	Total:	
Lunch:	Amount	Calories (kcal)
	Total:	

Snack:	Amount	Calories (kcal)
	Total:	

Dinner:	Amount	Calories (kcal)
	Total:	

Snack:	Amount	Calories (kcal)
	Total:	

Cups of Water: □□□□□□□□ **Servings of Fruits/Veggies:** □□□□□□□□

Exercise:	Duration	Calories (kcal) burned

DATE: Su Mo Tu We Th Fr Sa

Breakfast:	Amount	Calories (kcal)
	Total:	
Snack:	Amount	Calories (kcal)
	Total:	
Lunch:	Amount	Calories (kcal)
	Total:	

Snack:	Amount	Calories (kcal)
	Total:	

Dinner:	Amount	Calories (kcal)
	Total:	

Snack:	Amount	Calories (kcal)
	Total:	

Cups of Water: □□□□□□□□ **Servings of Fruits/Veggies:** □□□□□□□□

Exercise:	Duration	Calories (kcal) burned

DATE: Su Mo Tu We Th Fr Sa

Breakfast:	Amount	Calories (kcal)
	Total:	
Snack:	Amount	Calories (kcal)
	Total:	
Lunch:	Amount	Calories (kcal)
	Total:	

Snack:	Amount	Calories (kcal)
	Total:	

Dinner:	Amount	Calories (kcal)
	Total:	

Snack:	Amount	Calories (kcal)
	Total:	

Cups of Water: □□□□□□□□ **Servings of Fruits/Veggies:** □□□□□□□□

Exercise:	Duration	Calories (kcal) burned

DATE: Su Mo Tu We Th Fr Sa

Breakfast:	Amount	Calories (kcal)
	Total:	
Snack:	Amount	Calories (kcal)
	Total:	
Lunch:	Amount	Calories (kcal)
	Total:	

Snack:	Amount	Calories (kcal)
	Total:	

Dinner:	Amount	Calories (kcal)
	Total:	

Snack:	Amount	Calories (kcal)
	Total:	

Cups of Water: □□□□□□□□ **Servings of Fruits/Veggies:** □□□□□□□□

Exercise:	Duration	Calories (kcal) burned

DATE: Su Mo Tu We Th Fr Sa

Breakfast:	Amount	Calories (kcal)
	Total:	
Snack:	Amount	Calories (kcal)
	Total:	
Lunch:	Amount	Calories (kcal)
	Total:	

Snack:	Amount	Calories (kcal)
	Total:	

Dinner:	Amount	Calories (kcal)
	Total:	

Snack:	Amount	Calories (kcal)
	Total:	

Cups of Water: □□□□□□□□ **Servings of Fruits/Veggies:** □□□□□□□□

Exercise:	Duration	Calories (kcal) burned

DATE: Su Mo Tu We Th Fr Sa

Breakfast:	Amount	Calories (kcal)
	Total:	
Snack:	Amount	Calories (kcal)
	Total:	
Lunch:	Amount	Calories (kcal)
	Total:	

Snack:	Amount	Calories (kcal)
	Total:	

Dinner:	Amount	Calories (kcal)
	Total:	

Snack:	Amount	Calories (kcal)
	Total:	

Cups of Water: □□□□□□□□ **Servings of Fruits/Veggies:** □□□□□□□□

Exercise:	Duration	Calories (kcal) burned

DATE: Su Mo Tu We Th Fr Sa

Breakfast:	Amount	Calories (kcal)
	Total:	
Snack:	Amount	Calories (kcal)
	Total:	
Lunch:	Amount	Calories (kcal)
	Total:	

Snack:	Amount	Calories (kcal)
	Total:	

Dinner:	Amount	Calories (kcal)
	Total:	

Snack:	Amount	Calories (kcal)
	Total:	

Cups of Water: ☐☐☐☐☐☐☐☐ **Servings of Fruits/Veggies:** ☐☐☐☐☐☐☐☐

Exercise:	Duration	Calories (kcal) burned

DATE: Su Mo Tu We Th Fr Sa

Breakfast:	Amount	Calories (kcal)
	Total:	

Snack:	Amount	Calories (kcal)
	Total:	

Lunch:	Amount	Calories (kcal)
	Total:	

Snack:	Amount	Calories (kcal)
	Total:	

Dinner:	Amount	Calories (kcal)
	Total:	

Snack:	Amount	Calories (kcal)
	Total:	

Cups of Water: ☐☐☐☐☐☐☐☐ **Servings of Fruits/Veggies:** ☐☐☐☐☐☐☐☐

Exercise:	Duration	Calories (kcal) burned

DATE: Su Mo Tu We Th Fr Sa

Breakfast:	Amount	Calories (kcal)
	Total:	

Snack:	Amount	Calories (kcal)
	Total:	

Lunch:	Amount	Calories (kcal)
	Total:	

Snack:	Amount	Calories (kcal)
	Total:	

Dinner:	Amount	Calories (kcal)
	Total:	

Snack:	Amount	Calories (kcal)
	Total:	

Cups of Water: □□□□□□□□ **Servings of Fruits/Veggies:** □□□□□□□□

Exercise:	Duration	Calories (kcal) burned

DATE: **Su Mo Tu We Th Fr Sa**

Breakfast:	Amount	Calories (kcal)
	Total:	
Snack:	Amount	Calories (kcal)
	Total:	
Lunch:	Amount	Calories (kcal)
	Total:	

Snack:	Amount	Calories (kcal)
	Total:	

Dinner:	Amount	Calories (kcal)
	Total:	

Snack:	Amount	Calories (kcal)
	Total:	

Cups of Water: ☐☐☐☐☐☐☐☐ **Servings of Fruits/Veggies:** ☐☐☐☐☐☐☐☐

Exercise:	Duration	Calories (kcal) burned

NOTES ABOUT PERSONAL PROGRESS

Beginning Weight:	Ending Weight: